Body Butter Recipes

Proven Formula Secrets to Making All Natural Body Butters that Will Hydrate and Rejuvenate Your Skin

Jessica Jacobs

Jessica Jacobs

Table of Contents

Body Butter Recipes

Introduction

I want to thank you and congratulate you for downloading the book, *"Body Butter Recipes: Proven Formula Secrets to Making All Natural Body Butters that Will Hydrate and Rejuvenate Your Skin."*

This book contains all the information you will need to start making your own nurturing body butters. They are perfect for personal use and as gifts to your loved ones. This book is a comprehensive guide to discovering the world of rejuvenating homemade body butters that can be tailored to suit your skin type. Aside from their nourishing properties, the scents and oils used in the recipes are also therapeutic, and are proven to uplift your mood.

The reasons you will want to refer your family and friends to this book are:

- This book helps you to discover the enormous opportunities that nature gives to heal the largest human organ and body protector – your skin.

- This body butter book uses simple and straightforward language that makes for an interesting and easily understandable read.

- The ingredients in the body butter recipes are natural and non-toxic.

- It contains recipes that require only a couple of minutes to prepare.

- The book explains the proper method of choosing ingredients for body butters, and inspires you to create your own unique skincare product recipes.

- It shows the way to a healthy and well-nurtured skin. Supporting your skin with natural body butters helps keep it elastic and strong whether you are young or old.

- You have the power to take care of your skin without the damaging chemical substances that are found in many beauty products. Having great skin is actually in your hands!

- This book will make you realize that making skincare products at home is fun and easy. It really doesn't require much!

The ingredients in the natural body butters are not only healing for the skin; they also improve overall health and help you to reach mental balance. Your skin is the surface of your body, and it deserves the best care it can get. Now you can give it that care!

Thanks again for downloading this book, I hope you enjoy it!

Chapter 1: What Are Body Butters and Why You Should Make Your Own?

How much do you care for your skin? When you think of all the organs of your body – your heart, your lungs – how much importance do you place on your skin?

Most often, we tend to pay attention to skincare only when we notice that something is not right. When we start scratching because of dry or sensitive skin, develop stretch marks, or break out in rashes or allergies – these are the times when we realize how a big a role our skin plays in our wellbeing.

Skincare

Skincare has been around for millennia. The

ancient Egyptians and Romans were very particular about beauty, and developed many cosmetics and skincare products. However, our forebears used some ingredients that were not exactly safe, such as mercury and belladonna.

Thanks to modern science and research, harmful chemicals such as these have been banned from our skincare products. Now a wide variety of skincare products are available in any shop, and the choices are endless. Creams, lotions, moisturizers, healing salves: all have found a place on supermarket shelves, and so have body butters.

Body Butters

So, what are body butters, and how do they differ from other skincare products?

First, body butter is a type of skin moisturizer. Body butters are protective, nurturing, and intensely hydrating products with a thick consistency. Body lotions are mostly made of oils and water; body butters have less water and more oils, so they are basically really concentrated lotions.

Natural, homemade body butters are natural oils and butters mixed with other natural healing ingredients. And they can provide skincare that is up to ten times better than the most popular brands of commercially produced lotions!

Natural body butters are:

- Nurturing, softening skin moisturizers and protectors.

- Of thick consistency with concentrated healing properties.

- Made of natural fruit, seed and nut oils and butters with other natural ingredients such as essential oils, beeswax etc.

- Health and beauty aids that treat

symptoms and heal the entire body.

Your homemade body butters can provide what your skin needs, while nurturing it and protecting it from negative environmental influences.

Why Make Your Own Body Butters?

Making your own body butter is one of the smartest new trends in beauty and health care. It's a trend that has appeared and gained popularity in just the last couple of years, and definitely one whose time has come. Using your own body butter lets you take care of your skin and leaves you feeling safe and healthy at the same time.

Here is why you should make your own body butters:

- You know every ingredient that's inside,

and you know how the product has been made.

- You can design body butters that are 100% natural and have healing properties to nurture your skin and treat your skin conditions.

- You can make skincare products that not only heal your skin but also support your entire body.

- Making and using homemade body butters is a really fun and enjoyable process. You get to discover how things work and interact while gaining knowledge of the natural world and the human body.

The Problem with Commercial Skincare Products

Although we have access to a multitude of beauty products that claim to deliver superior skincare, pretty much all of them contain chemical and synthetic ingredients. Take a look at the back of your shampoo and body lotion containers and read the list of ingredients. Why are there so many chemicals in them?

Well, basically the chemicals in commercial skincare products are there to make them better smelling, longer lasting, and cheaper to manufacture. There is nothing wrong with that, as long as gorgeous aromas and lengthy shelf lives aren't acquired by adding harmful chemicals. Unfortunately, commercial skincare products are packed with many chemical additives that may do harm in the long term. Be honest with yourself – how many of the ingredients on the label of your body lotion do you really understand? How many of them are natural? How many of them really have any healing properties?

Aroma

To make commercial creams and lotions

smell nice, chemical aromas are added to them. This means that the "jasmine" in your jasmine lotion is very likely just a chemical that happens to smell like jasmine. The good news is that's not the way homemade body butters work. In our body butters, aromas come from essential oils derived from real flowers, and have strong healing properties.

Consistency

Natural body butters have a thicker consistency as there isn't much water used in making them. This thicker consistency means the body butter doesn't get absorbed into the skin very fast, which is why it is essential that the body butter be massaged all over the skin for it to penetrate into the organ's three layers.

Shelf Life

The shelf life of most homemade body

butters is about six months to one year. Commercial body butters, on the other hand, are made to last for several years – which would be impossible without chemical additives. This is the same truth behind the popularity of natural produce and vegetables nowadays: the life of a homegrown, natural tomato is relatively short, but it's packed with lots of vitamins and health supporters; the life of a chemically treated and cultivated tomato is a lot longer, but is there something for your health in it? Not really, because it's more about making money for the food producers, and less about health and well-being.

Ingredients

Many of the chemicals used in cosmetics are toxic and may cause harm to you. You might get smooth skin pretty fast, but at the same time you might be blocking pores and stimulating premature aging (or cancer growth, for cosmetics with unsafe ingredients). Don't do this to yourself! Know that there are healthy alternatives. Putting chemically-packed creams on your skin isn't skincare. Lathering on some natural body butters is.

If you don't understand what's written on the label of any product you are going to put on your skin – don't buy it. You have just one body given to you in this life, and although it regenerates itself, damaged cells won't regenerate without help. Make sure that skincare really means taking care of your skin, not just getting fast results and going through irreversible suffering later.

Chapter 2: Knowing Your Skin and Its Needs

That costume your body is dressed in is also the largest organ of your body, and it needs due care.

The functions of the skin include:

- Protecting the body from environmental influences and harmful microorganisms and substances;

- Regulating body temperature (thermoregulation);

- Receiving sensory information through millions of nerve endings;

- Producing vitamin D (yes, this happens

   right in your skin when it's exposed to sunlight);

- Acting as a barrier to keep the necessary nutrients inside the body and prevent excessive loss of fluids; and

- Absorption of oxygen and other essential nutrients, and storing water and lipids

Anatomy of Our Skin

Hair follicles, sweat glands and even fat are stored in our skin, which is built in three layers of cells:

The surface of the skin is called the epidermis, and it is the protective barrier that reacts to environmental influences and stops unwelcome substances from getting into the body. It also produces the skin pigment melanin, as well as keratin, which is the main substance for building the epidermis and ensuring the rigidity of the skin.

The layer right below the epidermis is the dermis. The dermis is the layer that's responsible for wrinkles and skin elasticity. This is where you can find blood vessels, oil glands, hair follicles, and sensory nerves. You can also find collagen and elastin here, which are also called the main ingredients in the fountain of youth. Collagen is a protein produced in the dermis which helps retain elasticity; however, negative environmental influences and aging reduce the production of collagen. The same happens with elastin: the skin gets loose and wrinkles appear as you age.

The deepest level of the skin is the subcutis or hypodermis. This skin layer is home to sweat glands, more collagen and fat. It's another body-protecting layer that conserves the heat of the body and keeps your skin fresh and rejuvenated.

The skin is affected from inside and outside, and it warrants special care if you want to keep it healthy, strong, and beautiful. First, it's important to keep the skin clean. Secondly, support your skin through healthy food choices and lifestyle; and third, nurture it outside with natural body butters.

Skin Conditions

It's great to have healthy, glowing skin. But as it ages, skin loses its ability to produce everything necessary for it to stay elastic and strong, and thus becomes susceptible to various skin conditions. Besides aging, skin problems are caused by unhealthy food choices, diseases, infections, viruses, dehydration, unhealthy environment, and so on.

Sunburn and skin cancer are not the only skin conditions caused by excessive sun exposure. Age spots, wrinkles, and loss of the skin's immune functions are on this list as well. Psoriasis and poor wound healing are not always related to genetics; they might be caused by using skincare products that contain alcohol, as these can actually dry out your skin. Cold weather is often the main cause for rosacea.

Being overweight often causes stretch marks and dermatitis, and cellulite appears on those with sedentary lifestyles.

There is a new field in medicine called psych dermatology, which states that many skin conditions, including vitiligo, psoriasis, hives and acne, are caused by stress and anxiety.

If you have a specific skin condition you want to get rid of, it's important to know where it comes from before you start treating it. Body butters that are tailored exactly for you could be the best healing agents for your particular skin needs.

A word of caution, though – body butters are not the lone solution for all skin problems. For example, will body butter solve your cellulite problem if your lifestyle remains sedentary? No. Will body butter give you healthy, glowing skin if you apply it without considering hygiene? No. There is no one wonder recipe to keep the skin young, soft, smooth, strong and glowing for your entire lifetime. You need to take care of your health inside and out, and be realistic when it comes to treating specific skin conditions.

Daily Skincare

What are the main rules for successful daily skincare?

First, keep it clean, but don't get too obsessed with cleanliness – that will damage your skin's natural ability to protect itself. What is too much cleanliness? Well, washing your body once a day is really enough. Twice is still fine, but more is already too much. Hands, of course, are an exception, because they get to touch everything that's around and gather a lot more microbes.

Besides bathing daily, you should moisturize your skin and take special care of exposed skin. Protect it from the sun with sunscreen. What else is important? Knowing your skin type and not applying too much makeup, for example, will certainly help.

Here are some tips to help you to get healthy skin:

- Respect your skin type and acknowledge that sensitive or dry skin definitely has different needs from elastic or oily skin.

- If you use makeup, don't overdo it. Use cosmetics that are natural or organic. Always remove your makeup as soon as you don't need it to let your skin breathe; don't wait until bedtime to get rid of it. Use natural makeup removers that can be simply applied on the skin with a cotton ball. Almond oil, for one, is all natural and does not irritate the eyes.

- There is no cream that will be better than oil-based body butter for daily moisturizing.

- The Skin Cancer Foundation warns that you are exposed to up to 40% of the sun's UV radiation even on cloudy days and when sitting in the shade. Make sure that your skin is always protected from UV radiation, not just when you are going to the beach. Also, even with sunscreen, avoid long periods of sun exposure. There are body butters you can prepare to use after sun exposure or even in place of sunscreen.

- Many experts say that oily skin is related to excess production of hormones in the body, so first think about balancing your hormones. Basically, oily skin is healthy, as the oil produced by the body is necessary for protection. Don't make the mistake of trying to get your skin too dry. If you have oily skin, body butters using an oil or butter base won't be suitable for you. Oily skin has to be moisturized as well, but with oil-free products.

- Don't use soap for washing dry and

  sensitive skin, as it can dry the skin out even more.

- Apply moisturizers on sensitive skin right after cleansing it. Avoid all chemically scented skincare products for sensitive skin as they could cause allergic reactions or irritation. If you want aromatic treatments, 100% pure essential oils added to homemade body butters will help.

- In winter, wear soft, natural fabrics close to your skin and moisturize your skin with body butters every night before sleep.

- Introduce body butters into your daily skincare routines. The best times for applying body butters are right after a bath or shower, or just before sleep.

- Your skin will get the most benefit from body butters if you use them just a few times per week, not necessarily every day.

Chapter 3: Body Butter Laboratory at Home: Equipment and Selecting the Ingredients

Creating your own body butters really doesn't require much. You don't have to be a pharmacist, and the ingredients are easy to find. What you need to do first is to educate yourself about the different ingredients and properties of body butters that will help you create what your skin needs. We will discuss the ingredients in the next chapters in this book. For now, let's talk about equipment.

Your laboratory is most likely going to be the kitchen, as you will need to melt ingredients over heat. It's a great experience to turn your kitchen into laboratory for creating skincare products. Don't worry, it's going to be easy and faster than cooking rice, and your body butters will be ready for use as soon as the mixture cools down.

Equipment

This is the equipment you will need:

Heatproof Containers

First, make sure that you have heatproof containers. To make body butters, the main process will be melting butters and oils and mixing them with other ingredients. This is usually done by putting ingredients in heatproof containers and setting them on low heat. Putting a heatproof bowl in a water bath – another heatproof container that's filled with water and set on heat, can also do it. Using a water bath for melting the ingredients will melt them more slowly and ensure you don't burn anything, as you usually don't bring them to boil. For beginners at making body butters, melting ingredients in a water bath is more convenient. Take note that the melting process is pretty fast, so you need to keep your attention on it.

Heatproof Gloves

You will deal with hot substances, so it might be useful to get some gloves and think of a safe, comfortable way to transfer them.

Thermometer, Measuring Cups & Spoons, Weighing Scale

For some recipes you find online, you will also need a scale for weighing butters and measuring cups or spoons for measuring oils. Many recipes do not require any of these – you can often just measure ingredients by eye. Also, melted ingredients usually do not need to reach any specific temperature; they are ready as soon as they have melted.

Mixer

To create whipped body butters that are softer and lighter you will need a mixer. This is not required for all recipes, and it's your choice whether to use it. It doesn't change the healing properties of the body butter, only the consistency.

Basically, that's it! Most likely, you already have the necessary equipment in your kitchen-laboratory.

Conversion Chart

Use this conversion chart to help you with liquid base oils and essential oils:

Essential Oil Drops	ml.	Teaspoons	Tablespoons	Cups	oz.
20	1				
100	5	1	¼		1/6
200	10	2	½		1/3
400	20	4	1		0.7
600	30	6	1 ½		1
1000	50	10	2 ½		1.7
2000	100	20	5		3.4
2500	125	25	6 ¼	½	4.

					2
5000	25 0	50	12 ½	1	8. 4

Selecting Ingredients for Your Body Butters

In the last chapter of this book, you will find several body butter recipes you can try to prepare at home for your personal needs. If you don't find one that is perfectly suitable for you, you can also try to invent your own oil and butter mixtures.

Here are the steps in selecting ingredients:

1. Know your skin and its needs. If you are not sure what your skin requires, visit a dermatologist who will help you understand what kind of skincare is suitable for you. If you don't have any specific skin condition and have normal,

healthy skin, any oil will help to support it, making it soft and glowing. If you have skin that suffers from one or more specific conditions, do not put something on your skin just because it is available. You must choose your ingredients wisely.

2. Educate yourself about the properties of herbs, oils, butters and other ingredients to enable you to choose them well according to the needs of your skin. We will take a look at the most popular body butter ingredients in the next chapters. Make sure that your skin can tolerate each of the ingredients you choose to mix together. You can do your own skin allergy tests by applying a small amount of each single ingredient on a small area of your body and waiting a few days to see if there is any reaction. If not, it's safe to mix them together in your body butters.

3. Purchase only 100% natural, high-quality

products. You will put them on your skin, and paying a bit more to get fully natural ingredients will pay back into your health. Added artificial chemicals and preservatives might do your skin more harm than good. Pharmacy-certified vendors are the places for purchasing the necessary ingredients. Always purchase fully closed containers in original packing to avoid fraud. Do not scent your body butters with artificially created aromas. To add aroma, always choose pure essential oils.

If any of the ingredients you want to use are difficult to find or seem too expensive, don't go for a lower-quality version of the same ingredient. It's better to look for an alternative ingredient with similar properties that's more available and affordable.

4. In creating your original body butter recipes, don't mix a dozen different

ingredients hoping to make a magical body butter that cures all possible skin issues. That won't happen, and you might go wrong. Go with 2-3 ingredients only. If you are using essential oils, do not add more than one, as the aroma could become too concentrated or strong. Make sure your body butter isn't more than 2% essential oil; just add a few drops.

5. Finally, check if you have all the necessary ingredients. Prepare them if needed (for example, infused oils), and step into the adventure of creating your own, original body butter.

Storing Your Homemade Body Butters

It would be a pity to damage your homemade treasure by storing it wrong. Body butters can be stored in plastic containers, but there might be a reaction between their oils and the plastic.

For example, essential oils can simply eat up plastic, although the content of essential oils in body butters isn't that high.

It would be better to store natural products in natural containers. The best are dark-colored glass containers or good old jars you can close tightly with lids. It's your choice, but the best option for storage is always the most natural one.

Chapter 4: Base Ingredients for Your Body Butters

The main ingredient in making body butters is the base, which is either butter or oil. These already have healing properties and the consistency of body butter. Other ingredients that are added to the base include essential oils, aloe vera gel, beeswax, and vitamin E.

There is such a wide variety of base butters and oils you can use to make body butters that we would need an encyclopedia to take a look at all of them. If you see a body butter recipe (you can look for them in the last chapter of this book), but can't find where to buy or order the mentioned oils or butters at an affordable price, you can also replace them with similar ones; you just have to know some of the basics.

Here are some of the most popular body butter base ingredients:

Almond Oil and Butter

It is rich with omega-9 and -6 fatty acids, vitamin E, and other active vitamins and minerals. It has calming properties and promotes healthy cholesterol levels in blood. It prevents aging, activates cell regeneration and soothes skin irritations. It is advised for oily, dry and tired skin. It helps in cellulite prophylaxis, smoothing wrinkles, treating eczema, and strengthening and toning skin. Besides the beneficial skin effects, it also activates brain functions.

This oil is generally safe for everyone; however, those who are allergic to nuts should use caution. It has light skin whitening effects – it doesn't make the skin pale, but gives it a healthy color.

Avocado Butter

It greatly assists regeneration and rejuvenation of skin tissue. It's packed with vitamins and minerals and is a great nutrient and moisturizer for dry and mature skin. Age spots, sunburn and eczema can be treated with the help of avocado butter. It also contains omega-3, can protect the skin from UV radiation, and rejuvenates aging skin by erasing wrinkles. This butter is especially advised for aging skin.

Cocoa Butter

It is called cocoa butter because it is extracted from cocoa beans, the main ingredient in chocolate. Cocoa butter melts at body temperature, so it's easy to apply on the skin. Skin absorbs products with cocoa butter quickly, and it's a great moisturizer that keeps skin soft and hydrated. It also prevents stretch marks for pregnant women, and is good for treating psoriasis, eczema, and dry, rough and damaged skin. It also provides collagen to the skin, protecting the skin from aging by restoring its elasticity.

Coconut Oil

This oil, which has a solid consistency at room temperature and melts when warmed, seems more like butter than oil. Its lipid content is really close to that of human skin, so this oil gets absorbed pretty fast, doesn't block pores, and is suitable for any type of skin. It's so gentle that it can also be used on teenagers, kids and infants. It's rich in vitamins A, B and E, calcium and iron, and is widely used for natural skincare. It's well known as the best protector against environmental and climate influences, and can be used as a natural sunscreen that protects from UV radiation. Coconut oil also soothes sunburns and prevents skin from aging by keeping it elastic. As it's absorbed easily, it gets into the deepest layers of the skin. It is good for treating dry skin, psoriasis and skin irritation, and for nurturing and strengthening skin.

Evening Primrose Oil

This is probably one of the cosmetic oils most celebrated by women. It not only helps to rejuvenate skin and prevent aging, but also helps to ease PMS, chronic headache, symptoms of menopause, and joint pain. It's one of the few oils that contain high concentrations of GLA (gamma-linoleic acid), which is essential for every organ of the human body – that's probably one of the main reasons why this oil can provide such a great healing benefit. It helps to balance hormones, treats skin inflammations, dermatitis, psoriasis and eczema, and it improves skin elasticity and blood circulation. Evening primrose is a great support when taking care of dry and mature skin.

Grape seed Oil

Grape seed oil has a very subtle scent that is almost unperceivable when you mix it with other ingredients. It has high biologic activity and contains antioxidants that slow down the process of cell aging. Grape seed oil contains linoleic acid and vitamin E, making it a great moisturizer that prevents skin from drying out, gives the skin a fresh look, rejuvenates skin that has suffered from sun and wind exposure, and prevents skin from forming wrinkles. It gets absorbed fast and is suitable for all skin types, but especially for skin that lacks hydration.

Jojoba Oil

This is one of the rare oils that are advised for treating oily skin. It prevents skin dehydration, and soothes and softens the skin, preventing wrinkles. The skin absorbs it pretty fast, and it also has a pleasant aroma. It is an anti-inflammatory skin moisturizer that can help restore the balance of sebum levels produced by the human body.

Kokum Butter

It is made from the Garcinia tree that grows in India. This butter contains a bucket of minerals and vitamins that help restore tired skin and improve its regeneration, supporting skin elasticity. It has a pretty hard consistency, but makes a great skincare product when mixed with oils. It soothes and nurtures damaged and dry skin, and supports and improves the natural protective barrier of the body.

Mango Butter

It comes from the tropical rainforest where it

has been used traditionally as a natural skincare product for ages. It soothes the skin, helps to keep it elastic and toned, protects against UV radiation, and is a great moisturizer. An effective treatment for dry skin, skin rashes and peeling, it also eases muscle aches and tension, and decreases signs of aging.

Olive Oil

It has antibacterial properties and nurturing, calming characteristics with positive effects on the digestive and nervous system. Due to its content of antioxidants and vitamin E, it's a good skin protector that helps to keep the skin elastic, treat stretch marks and prevent aging. This is especially suitable for dry and sensitive skin. Due to the anti-cancer properties this oil has, it's advised to use skincare products containing olive oil right after sun exposure. Skin absorbs this oil pretty slowly, so mostly it's used in small amounts in combination with larger quantities of other oils/butters.

Shea Butter

Rich in vitamins A and E, this butter made from the seeds of the Shea tree is a great moisturizer that treats skin allergies, blemishes, wounds, eczema, dermatitis, insect bites, rough skin, skin cracks and sunburns. It almost immediately stops itchiness, is great for dry skin and is ideal for after shaving. It's one of the most popular body butter base ingredients and is even called the "skin's best friend" due to its healing and skin-softening properties.

Chapter 5: Herb-Infused Oils

As you get closer to creating your own body butters, you can also consider including herb-infused oils in the list of ingredients. Infused oils can be applied to skin alone or mixed into body butters as an addition to the base, or even as the base by themselves.

Infused Oils vs. Essential Oils

Infused oils are carrier or base oils that have gained additional properties from infusion with fresh or dried herbs. These are not pure oils, nor essential oils. Many herbs offer truly great healing properties, but they can't be extracted to get oil or essential oil – and in this case infusions are a great way to use the herb's properties for skincare products. For example, there is no oil that is produced from calendula, but you probably have seen calendula oil for sale – that's infused oil that has been made by soaking the herb in a base oil.

Herbs also add aroma to the oil of infusion. It would be easier to add a few drops of essential oil to body butters, but you cannot always find essential oils of specific plants. Essential oils are also very concentrated herbal extracts and may simply be too strong for some people, while infused oils contain lower concentrations of plant extract.

Natural vs. Commercial Infused Oils

The problem with commercially produced infused oils is that you cannot always see from the labels what kind of carrier oil has actually been used to deliver the herbal properties. If you are allergic to nuts, it would be a pity if you inadvertently used calendula oil that had been made on a walnut or almond oil base. The solution is making your own herbal infusions with base oils of your choice.

Popular Herbs for Infusion

The most popular herbs for making infused oils for skincare are calendula, lavender, rosemary, peppermint and chamomile. However, many other herbs can be infused as well. If you know the healing properties of an herb and are sure that's what your skin needs (or your doctor says you can benefit from it), go ahead and make your own herbal infusion of it to use for making body butters.

The carrier in which to soak the herb can be any of the previously mentioned oils or butters, although it's obviously much easier to do it with oils than butters.

How to Infuse Oils at Home

Preparing your own herb-infused oils isn't difficult; it just takes time.

Here are two ways to prepare herb-infused oils: cold infusions and heat infusions. You will get the same results either way, so choose the one that seems more convenient for you. Cold infusions are suitable only for oils with liquid consistency, but solid butters or oils that are solid at room temperature can be infused only by the heat infusion method.

Cold Infusion

Ingredients and equipment:

- Fresh or dried herb you want to extract

- Carrier oil you want to infuse

- A glass jar with tightfitting lid

- Cheesecloth

Steps:

1. Prepare herbs by crushing or plucking them, but do not powder them (if using dried herbs). Don't use freshly washed herbs or wet equipment to avoid the inclusion of water in the infusion process.

2. Put herbs in the jar and pour enough oil to cover the herbs.

3. Close the jar with a lid and place it in a warm spot, as the heat is what promotes herb extraction. If you are using a dark-colored jar, you can leave it on a sunny windowsill, but if it's a light or transparent jar do not put it in direct sunlight to avoid losing the healing properties. Direct sunlight destroys some of the essential active ingredients.

4. Leave the jar in a warm place for 4-6 weeks. Check and gently shake the jar every few days to make sure herbs are

well covered in oil and promote release of herbal properties.

5. After 4-6 weeks, strain the oil through cheesecloth into a clean container to remove the herb pieces. The infused oil is now ready to be used.

Hot Infusion

Ingredients and equipment:

- Fresh or dried herb you want to extract

- Carrier oil you want to infuse

- Crockpot or stove, saucepan and heatproof bowl

- Cheesecloth

Steps:

1. Put a saucepan filled with water on the lowest heat and place a heatproof bowl inside it, making a water bath. If you are

using a crockpot, put it on the lowest heat.

2. Add herbs to the bowl and pour the oil to cover them (or add the ingredients to the crockpot).

3. Leave it to simmer on the lowest heat for about 5-8 hours, stirring every hour. Don't let it boil or cook, and don't cover it with a lid to let the excess water evaporate.

4. After it's done, leave the mixture to cool down.

5. When the mixture has cooled, strain it through cheesecloth to remove all herb pieces from the oil. The infused oil is now ready to use.

For beginners, the cold infusion method is the safest as the heat infusion method is a very technical process; accidentally burning or boiling the mixture loses all its herbal properties.

Chapter 6: Popular Ingredients Added to Body Butter Base

These are ingredients that are usually added to melted oil and butter mixtures to increase or add healing properties and/or scents.

Aloe Vera Gel

Native Americans called the aloe vera plant the "Wand of the Heavens", and it really seems to be a wonderful helper when it comes to skincare. Liquid gel from fresh leaves of the aloe vera plant treats acne, helps to heal sunburns, and protects the skin from the damaging effects of intensive sun exposure. It also relieves rashes and improves skin tissue renewal. It heals dry skin, blisters, rashes, skin irritations and bruises, scars and stretch marks, psoriasis, rosacea, eczema and skin allergies. Aloe vera gel is also known to decrease dark skin spots, and even helps in erasing wrinkles. It's a moisturizer that's quickly absorbed by skin.

Pure, natural aloe vera gel doesn't have a very long shelf life, and you should keep it in the refrigerator. If you prepare body butter with aloe vera gel, you should keep it in the refrigerator as well, and make only a small amount, as its shelf life is only about two months.

Beeswax

Beeswax is a popular ingredient for making healing salves and balms, but not so popular for body butters due to its hard consistency. Usually it's not mixed with butters (as they already give the preparations a solid consistency), but it is a great addition to mixed oils that take on a solid consistency when cooling down. Beeswax is also a great thickening agent for body butters.

Besides changing the consistency of mixed oils, it also offers healing properties. First, it makes a protective barrier on the skin surface. No worries, it's not a visible barrier, and it doesn't block pores. It's a natural barrier that allows the skin to breathe. It has antibacterial and skin-softening properties, and it also protects the skin from dehydration and negative environmental influences.

Essential Oils

Most body butters are made with 100% pure essential oils due to their healing benefits and positive effects for the entire body. Essential oils are concentrated plant extracts and thus have very strong aromas. They contain natural active ingredients with a wide variety of healing properties for all types of skin. They can uplift our mood and even heal internal organs. They are the main treatments used in aromatherapy, an ancient healing method that is a big part of alternative medicine nowadays.

Essential oils work in two ways – through inhaling the aromas to allow natural chemicals to travel to the brain, or by massage to get them into each cell of the skin. Ultimately, essential oils heal the body on two levels – physical and mental.

There are a great number of essential oils that can treat different health issues in different ways, but not all of them are popular body butter ingredients as their strengths and aromas differ. If you use essential oils extensively, you should have a background in aromatherapy. Here are the most popular essential oils for homemade skincare preparations along with their healing properties:

Chamomile

It is a gentle essential oil for every skin type that can be used at any age. It heals skin rashes and relieves allergies; especially suitable for dry skin.

Frankincense

It is an essential oil with a spirit-uplifting scent that relieves stress and encourages a meditative mood. It has anti-depression properties. Also on the mental level, this essential oil relieves stress and anxiety, helping you to gain and keep emotional balance. On the physical level this oil is well-known for use with mature skin as it prevents aging, helps to get rid of wrinkles, heals wounds, alleviates allergic skin reactions, eases headache and is also a great support for the body's immune system.

Geranium

It is another essential oil that relieves nervous tension and stress, helping to keep emotional balance. It heals dry and sensitive skin.

Lavender

If there is one essential oil that should be in everyone's medicine chest, this is the one. It can be used for all skin types and offers a great variety of healing properties. Lavender heals burns and sunburns, cuts and wounds, blisters and insect bites. It eases allergies, headaches, stress and emotional imbalances, treats insomnia and encourages skin tissue renewal, and that's just a small part of the issues that can be relieved and healed with the help of lavender essential oil.

Lemongrass

An essential oil with a sweet, fresh aroma that helps for varicose veins, muscle strains and water retention. It has mood-uplifting, antiseptic and anti-fungal properties.

Patchouli

A kind of oil with antiseptic and anti-inflammatory properties that are especially suitable for dry and mature skin. It protects skin from UV radiation, improves skin elasticity, and has been successfully used as an additional treatment for obesity, cellulite and water retention.

Peppermint

A truly refreshing and cooling essential oil that relieves pain and muscle tension, improves mental performance, strengthens the immune system and is also an antidepressant. It is advised to use it in cooling skincare products for oily skin.

Rose

This oil is relatively expensive, but also effective and highly appreciated for skincare. It prevents aging and scarring, heals wounds, protects against sunburn, helps to smooth wrinkles and encourages emotional balance.

Sandalwood

An antiseptic essential oil that helps to heal skin tumors, rashes and infections, is especially suitable for dry skin, protects against UV radiation, and supports skin tissue regeneration.

Ylang-Ylang

This is an essential oil with a very sweet aroma that treats psoriasis, eczema and acne. It prevents aging, regulates hormonal balance and encourages a feeling of well being.

Of course, there are many other essential oils that are used for body butters, but these are just the basics. If you are not experienced in using essential oils, do not add more than one to homemade body butter recipes to avoid unwelcome skin reactions.

As essential oils are extremely concentrated plant extracts, you will need only a few drops to add the healing properties to your body butter. Also, make sure you don't add more than 2% of essential oil content in your body butters, and not more than 1% if you have very sensitive skin or are planning to use this butter on large areas of your body.

For example, if you are making 5 ml (1 teaspoon) of mixture add only 1 drop of essential oil to reach 1% of it in the mixture. For 10 ml (2 teaspoons) – 2 drops, for 100 ml (5 tablespoons) – 20 drops of essential oil and so on.

Honey

Honey is another remedy known and used for

centuries to treat different health conditions. Mostly, of course, honey is ingested, but it can also be applied on the skin. It is rich in nutrients, and has antibacterial and antioxidant properties. Due to these characteristics, honey helps to prevent aging. It's a great moisturizer that keeps the skin well-hydrated, and helps it regenerate to stay soft and youthful.

Vitamin E Oil

It's an effective remedy for premature aging that is caused by unhealthy lifestyle and environmental influences. Vitamin E oil is widely used in many skincare products and homemade body butters. It blocks the damage caused by free radicals, promotes the skin cell regeneration and growth process, and increases the body's natural production of collagen. This means that this oil helps to prevent aging, keeps skin elastic, hydrated and strong, removes dark skin spots and heals scars.

Although vitamin E oil sounds like a magical remedy, do not overuse it as it can be hard for the skin to deal with large quantities. If it's in all your skincare products you may end up with an allergic reaction. Always make sure you use the most natural form of vitamin E oil you can get. As its popularity has increased, inferior oils are often sold in an attempt to cash in on the trend. Synthetic forms of vitamin E oil will not be as effective as the natural ones. If you can't find natural oil, simply skip this ingredient - your body butters will have healing, moisturizing and rejuvenating properties anyway.

Chapter 7: Simple Body Butter Recipes

Here you will find different interesting and easy-to-make body butter recipes to use for making your own butters. It will also help you to understand the process and provide a foundation for your creativity in case you are looking to create your own recipes. For beginners, try any of these recipes!

Whipped Aloe Vera Body Butter

Ingredients:

- 3 tablespoons Shea butter

- 3 tablespoons aloe vera gel

- 2 tablespoons coconut oil

- 1 teaspoon of jojoba oil

- Optional: 10 drops of essential oil of your choice

Steps:

1. Combine Shea butter and coconut oil and melt them.

2. Stir to combine well; remove from the heat once they liquefy. Leave to cool down, but not so cool as to return to solid consistency.

3. When the coconut-Shea butter mixture is starting to solidify, add aloe vera gel, jojoba oil and essential oil. Use a mixer to combine them all and whip. It should take about 12-15 minutes to achieve an airy consistency.

4. With a wooden spoon, transfer your body butter to a jar container. Store in a cool, dry place to avoid melting and loss of the light consistency.

Useful tip: As it contains aloe vera, store this body butter in a refrigerator. Also, make sure you use it within two months as aloe vera doesn't have a long shelf life.

Simple Moisturizing Butter

Ingredients:

- 4 tablespoons coconut oil

- 4 tablespoons Shea butter

- 2 tablespoons Grape seed oil

- 1 teaspoon beeswax pastilles (or grated beeswax)

- Optional: a few drops of essential oil of your choice to add aroma

Steps:

1. Combine all ingredients and melt them.

2. When they have melted, stir them and remove from heat. If using essential oils, add them and stir at this point.

3. Transfer the mixture to a storage container while it's still warm, because it will solidify after cooling down.

Useful tip: Pour this body butter into small containers, for example, ice cube trays. You can later use one cube at a time for ease of use and application.

Rose Body Butter "Almost Royal"

Ingredients:

- ½ cup almond oil

- ½ cup rosewater

- 1 tablespoon of beeswax pastilles or grated beeswax

- 15 drops of rose essential oil

Steps:

1. Melt beeswax, and when it's half melted, slowly pour in almond oil.

2. When the beeswax has melted, making a smooth mass with the almond oil, remove it from the heat and add rosewater and rose essential oil.

3. After stirring to combine well, pour this liquid consistency butter into a container for storage.

Useful tip: This body butter doesn't get a very thick consistency, so it can be stored in a container with a pump dispenser. Due to the water content in this product, it's advised to keep it in the refrigerator.

Gentle Care for Aging Skin

Ingredients:

- ½ cup of evening primrose oil

- ½ Grape seed oil

- 10 drops of lavender essential oil

- 10 drops of frankincense essential oil

Steps:

1. Mix together all the ingredients.

2. Pour into storage containers.

Useful Tip: As you don't add butters in this recipe, you can keep this mixture in a glass bottle. If you want to get a thicker and more butter-like consistency, melt any of the previously mentioned butters and add to the mixture. For example, avocado butter will be a great addition to this product for mature and aging skin.

Stretch Mark Eraser

Ingredients:

- ½ cup cocoa butter

- ½ cup Shea butter

- 3 tablespoons almond oil

- 3 tablespoons olive oil

- 10 drops of lavender essential oil

- 10 drops of geranium essential oil

- 10 drops of patchouli essential oil

Steps:

1. Melt together cocoa and Shea butters. When they have almost completely melted, slowly add olive and almond oils.

2. When everything has melted, making a smooth mass, remove from heat and stir in essential oils.

3. Transfer to storage containers.

Simple Protector Against UV Radiation

Ingredients:

- 1 cup coconut oil

- 20-40 drops of patchouli essential oil

- Optional: 1 teaspoon vitamin E oil

Steps:

1. Combine all ingredients in a mixing bowl (add coconut oil without melting it).

2. Whisk with a mixer for about 10 minutes until it gets an airy consistency.

3. With a spoon, transfer the body butter to a storage container.

Useful tip: Store the body butter in the refrigerator or any other cool place to avoid it melting and losing its light consistency.

Rejuvenating Calendula Body Butter

Ingredients:

- ½ cup calendula infused oil
- 4 tablespoons Shea butter
- 3 tablespoons kokum butter

Steps:

1. Melt together Shea and kokum butters.
2. When they have almost fully melted, slowly add calendula infused oil.
3. Stir mixture to combine well and remove from heat.
4. Pour into storage container.

Useful tip: You can also whip it using a mixer before it has fully cooled and before transferring to a storage container.

Refreshing Body Butter for Hot Summer Days

Ingredients:

- ½ cup coconut oil

- ½ cup aloe vera gel

- 3 tablespoons beeswax pastilles or grated beeswax

- 10-20 drops of peppermint essential oil

Steps:

1. Melt together coconut oil and beeswax.

2. When they are melted, remove from the heat and stir in the rest of the ingredients.

3. Transfer to storage container.

Useful tip: You can also let the butter cool down and then whisk it by mixer to get a lighter consistency before transferring to a storage container. If whisked, keep this body butter in the refrigerator.

Calming Lavender Body Butter

Ingredients:

- 5 tablespoons coconut oil

- 2 tablespoons olive oil

- 2 tablespoons beeswax pastilles or grated beeswax

- 1 teaspoon honey

- 10 drops lavender essential oil

Steps:

1. Heat and melt coconut and olive oils, beeswax and honey all together.

2. Stir them to combine, and when they make a smooth mass, remove from heat.

3. Add lavender essential oil into warm

mixture and pour into storage containers.

Tropical Body Butter

Ingredients:

- 5 tablespoons mango butter

- 4 tablespoons cocoa butter

- 20 drops of ylang-ylang essential oil

Steps:

1. Combine mango and coconut butters and melt them.

2. Once melted and forming a smooth mass, remove from heat and add essential oil.

3. Transfer into storage container.

Useful tip: Pour this body butter in small containers, for example, ice cube trays. You can later use one cube at a time for ease of use and application.

Whipped Peppermint Body Butter

Ingredients

- 1 cup of coconut oil

- 1 cup of cocoa butter

- 1 cup of Shea butter

- 1 cup of almond oil

- 2 tsp. of vitamin E oil

- 4-8 drops of peppermint essential oil

Steps

1. Place a pot over low heat and add the coconut oil, Shea butter and cocoa butter. Keep stirring till they melt and combine together. Then remove from heat.

2. Add in the sweet almond oil, vitamin E oil and peppermint.

3. Place the mixture in the fridge for a couple of hours so that it becomes a little firm.

4. Then whip the mixture to your desired consistency.

5. Scoop it all into a jar and you can use it for the next few months. If the consistency is lost due to hot weather, just whip it again.

Chocolate Orange Body Butter

Ingredients

- 1 cup of coconut oil

- 1 cup of cocoa butter

- 40-60 drops of orange essential oil

Steps

1. Place a saucepan on low heat and melt the coconut oil with the cocoa butter. Keep stirring till they mix well.

2. Transfer the above mixture to a mixing bowl and add the orange oil to it.

3. Refrigerate the mixture till it is firm but not hard.

4. Use a hand mixer or a whipping appliance to thoroughly whip the butter into a light and fluffy consistency.

5. Scoop the delicious-smelling butter into some glass jars and store for use. Keep it tightly covered when not in use.

Mint Eucalyptus Body Butter

Ingredients

- 7 tbsp. of cocoa butter

- ½ cup of coconut oil

- 7 tbsp. of Shea butter

- 1 tbsp. of carrier oil

- 2 tsp. of castor oil

- 11 drops of eucalyptus essential oil

- 4 drops of peppermint essential oil

Steps

1. Melt the cocoa butter, Shea butter and coconut oil in a pot over medium heat. When it is soft and well infused, transfer the mixture to a bowl.

2. To this mixture, add the castor oil, carrier oil, and eucalyptus and peppermint essential oils. Stir well. Keep the bowl in the fridge till the mixture holds together firmly.

3. Now whip up the mixture till it is soft and fluffy. Use a hand mixer or a whipping appliance.

4. Transfer the whipped body butter into a glass jar and use as required.

Rosemary Mint Body Butter

Ingredients

- 4 tbsp. of cocoa butter

- 7 tbsp. of Shea butter

- 22 drops of spearmint essential oil

- 12 drops of rosemary essential oil

Steps

1. Use a double broiler to melt your cocoa and Shea butter together. Stir continuously over low heat till they melt.

2. Cool the mixture in a bowl and place it in the freezer for about 20 minutes.

3. Then use a whisker to whip it to a thick and fluffy consistency. Add the spearmint and rosemary essential oils at this point.

4. Keep whipping for a little while more to get soft, whipped body butter.

5. Store this in a jar and use it within a couple of months. Make sure your storage space is fairly cool; this mixture will melt if the temperature gets too warm.

Mango Citrus Body Butter

Ingredients

- 1 tsp. jojoba wax

- 1 tbsp. of cocoa butter

- 2 tbsp. of Shea butter

- 1 tbsp. of mango butter

- 1 tsp. of almond oil

- 1 tsp. of vitamin E

- 10 drops of lime essential oil

- 5 drops of orange essential oil

Steps

1. Place the jojoba wax, cocoa butter and mango butter over a double broiler to melt. Use low heat and stir constantly.

2. Remove from heat and add the almond oil and vitamin E while it is still hot. Let it cool a bit before adding the essential oils.

3. Stir the mixture thoroughly so that all the ingredients are well blended.

4. Scoop it into glass jars and store.

Argan Mango Body Butter

Ingredients

- 3 tbsp. of beeswax

- 2 tbsp. of mango butter

- 1 tbsp. of argan oil

- 2 tbsp. of cocoa butter

- 2 tbsp. of apricot kernel oil

Steps

1. Melt the beeswax, cocoa butter and mango butter over low heat in a pan. Keep stirring and melt till they combine.

2. Pour this into a mixing bowl and add the argan oil and apricot kernel oil.

3. Stir them all together and refrigerate for a while till the mixture is firm.

4. Use a hand mixer to whip it into a soft, creamy consistency.

5. Scoop it into your containers and use whenever you want. Keep it in a cool place or the consistency will be lost.

Chocolate and Lavender Body Butter

Ingredients

- 1 cup of coconut oil

- 1/3 cup of clear agave nectar

- 1 tbsp. of vanilla powder

- 1/3 cup of cacao powder

- 2-3 drops of lavender essential oil

Steps

1. Melt the coconut oil over low heat and pour into a bowl.

2. Add the agave, vanilla, cacao and lavender essential oil.

3. Pour this into a blender and run till they all blend well.

4. Cool this mixture in the fridge till it sets well.

5. Scoop it into jars and store in a cool place till you need to use.

Vanilla Bean Body Butter

Ingredients

- 2 cups of cocoa butter

- 1 cup of sweet almond oil

- 1 cup of coconut oil

- 2 vanilla beans

Steps

1. Take a double broiler and melt the cocoa butter and coconut oil over low heat. Then keep it aside to cool for a while.

2. Grind the vanilla beans using a food processor.

3. Now add the ground vanilla beans and

sweet almond oil into the cocoa and coconut mixture.

4. Stir these together well and keep in the fridge for about half an hour till firm.

5. Now whip the mixture into soft and fluffy body butter.

6. Scoop this into a glass jar and store in a cool place till you want to use it.

Lemon Cream Body Butter

Ingredients

- 12 tbsp. of coconut oil

- ½ cup of cocoa butter

- 2 tbsp. of vitamin E oil

- 1 tsp. of lemon essential oil

Steps

1. Place a saucepan over low heat and put the coconut oil and cocoa butter into it. Melt them together and remove from heat.

2. Add the vitamin E and lemon essential oil to this mixture.

3. Cool the mixture for a couple of hours.

4. Then pour it into containers to store for future use.

5. Use with a couple of months.

Lemongrass Toning Butter

Ingredients

- 100 g of cocoa butter

- 40 drops of lemongrass essential oil

- 50 g of almond oil

- 50 g of jojoba oil

Steps

1. Melt the cocoa butter over low heat in a saucepan.

2. Transfer this into a mixing bowl and add the lemongrass, almond and jojoba oil.

3. Whisk it up with a whipping appliance and scoop into a jar for storage.

Orange and Poppy Seed Scrubbing Butter

Ingredients

- 100 g cocoa butter

- 1 tbsp. of cocoa powder

- 30 drops of orange essential oil

- 2 tsp. of sea salt

- 1 tbsp. of poppy seeds

Steps

1. Use a double broiler to melt the cocoa butter. Then remove from heat and pour into a mixing bowl.

2. Add the orange essential oil and cocoa powder and mix well with a spatula. Allow it to cool for a while.

3. Then add the sea salt and poppy seeds. Mix evenly so that all the ingredients are well distributed.

4. Scoop your scrubbing butter into jars and keep in the bathroom to use while bathing.

Winter Body Butter

Ingredients

- 4 tbsp. of candelilla wax

- 100 g of meadowfoam seed oil

- 100 g of olive oil

- 120 g of avocado butter

- 10 g of winter white fragrance oil

Steps

1. Melt the candelilla wax, meadowfoam and olive oil in a double broiler.

2. Keep stirring for a couple of minutes till they mix well.

3. Take the mixture off the heat and pour it into a bowl.

4. Add avocado butter while the mixture is still hot.

5. Now add the winter white fragrance oil and stir well.

6. Pour it into glass jars and leave it to set.

7. Your winter balm is ready!

Coffee Body Butter

Ingredients

- 500 g of coffee butter

- 30 g of rice bran oil

- 15 g of tamanu oil

- 20 drops of vanilla essential oil

- 10 drops of sweet almond oil

Steps

1. Whip the coffee butter using a stand mixer for a minute to soften it.

2. Add the rice bran oil, tamanu oil, almond oil and vanilla oil to this. Keep whisking till the oils blend into the butter well.

3. Then whisk on high for a while till the consistency is light and fluffy.

4. Scoop this into jars and use whenever you want, but within the year.

Coconut and Plum Body Butter

Ingredients

- 50 g of coconut cream oil

- 50 g of cocoa butter

- 25 g of plum kernel oil

- 12 g of carnauba wax

- 2 tsp. of plum jojoba wax beads

Steps

1. Melt the cocoa butter, coconut oil, carnauba wax and plum wax over a double broiler on medium heat and stir well till they have melted completely.

2. Then add the plum kernel oil and remove from heat.

3. Place this over a bowl of cold water and whip till it thickens.

4. When the mixture has thickened and reached a fluffy consistency, scoop it into your containers. Let it set for a couple of hours.

5. You can use this butter for the next 2-3 months.

Macadamia Nut and Vanilla Body Butter

Ingredients

- 30 g of macadamia nut butter

- 10 g of vanilla essential oil

- 6 g of beeswax

Steps

1. Take a double broiler and place it over medium heat. Melt the macadamia nut butter and beeswax in this till they combine.

2. Take it off the heat and pour into a bowl. Add the vanilla oil and stir thoroughly.

3. Pour it into glass jars and let it set for some time.

4. Use within a couple of months.

Bronzing Body Butter

Ingredients

- 2 cups of Shea butter

- 1 cup of coconut oil

- 1 cup of jojoba oil

- 4 tbsp. of cocoa powder

- 2 tsp. of vitamin E oil

- 15 drops of peppermint essential oil

Steps

1. Melt the Shea butter and coconut oil over

a double broiler on low heat. When they melt completely, remove from heat and keep it aside to cool for a while.

2. Then add the jojoba oil, cocoa powder, vitamin E and peppermint essential oil. Use as much cocoa powder as you deem required for your skin.

3. Mix it all well and keep in the freezer till it is firm.

4. Once you remove it from the freezer, whip up the mixture to a smooth consistency till peaks form.

5. Scoop it into glass jars for storage.

Magnesium Body Butter

Ingredients

- 1 cup of magnesium flakes

- 6 tbsp. of boiling water

- ½ cup of virgin coconut oil

- 4 tbsp. of beeswax

- 6 tbsp. of Shea butter

Steps

1. Dissolve the magnesium flakes in the boiling water till you get a thick liquid. Let it cool down.

2. Use a double broiler to melt the coconut oil, beeswax and Shea butter. Keep stirring over medium heat till they all combine well. Remove from heat and let it cool.

3. Pour this into a mixing bowl and blend slowly using a hand mixer.

4. Slowly add in the magnesium liquid while whipping the mixture. Do this till it is all well blended.

5. Keep the mixture in the fridge for a while and then whip again to a smooth, buttery

consistency.

6. Scoop it into mason jars for later use.

7. Store in a cool place or the fridge for best results.

Strawberry Body Butter

Ingredients

- 50 g of Shea butter

- 1 tsp. of jojoba oil

- 1 tsp. of apricot oil

- 25 g of coconut oil

- ½ tsp. of strawberry food flavoring

- 2 drops of red food coloring

Steps

1. Melt the Shea butter and coconut oil in a double broiler over low heat.

2. Remove from heat and pour into a mixing bowl.

3. Add the rest of the ingredients and mix well using a spatula or hand mixer.

4. Scoop your yummy strawberry butter into mason jars and use!

Tangerine Shea Body Butter

Ingredients

- 60 g of Shea butter

- 25 g of coconut oil

- 2 tbsp. of macadamia nut oil

- 2 tsp. of jojoba oil

- 2 tsp. of sweet almond oil

- 2 tsp. of organic sunflower oil

- 10 drops of tangerine essential oil

Steps

1. Use a double boiler over medium heat to melt the Shea butter with coconut oil.

2. Remove the mixture from heat once it is completely melted.

3. Add the macadamia, jojoba, almond and sunflower oil. Mix it well.

4. Pour in the tangerine oil drops and whisk with a hand mixer.

5. Scoop this into jars and use anytime!

Green Tea Body Butter

Ingredients

- 4 tbsp. of beeswax

- ½ cup of virgin coconut oil

- ½ cup of grape seed oil

- ½ cup of oats made with hot water

- ½ cup of strong green tea

- 5 drops of rosemary oil

Steps

1. Melt the beeswax, coconut oil and grape seed oil using a double broiler. Let it cool once it is completely melted.

2. Mix the oats and green tea together in a glass.

3. Pour the oil mixture into a mixing bowl and blend well. Slowly pour the oat and green tea mixture into this.

4. Keep blending till you get the required consistency. Then add in the rosemary essential oil.

5. Scoop the cream into jars and keep it in a cool place. This body butter keeps best at

lower temperatures, so you might want to refrigerate it during the summer.

Cinnamon Body Butter

Ingredients

- 50 g of coconut oil

- 25 g of cocoa butter

- 25 g of Shea butter

- 15 drops of cinnamon oil

- A small cinnamon stick

Steps

1. Melt the coconut oil and Shea butter over medium heat. Keep stirring and then turn off the heat and let it cool for a while.

2. Then add the cinnamon oil and whip the mixture to a soft and fluffy consistency

using a hand mixer.

3. Grate the cinnamon stick with a cheese grater and mix it in.

4. Scoop this into jars; keep them tightly closed between uses.

Melon Body Butter

Ingredients

- 50 g of Shea butter

- 1 tsp. of jojoba oil

- 4 tbsp. of coconut oil

- 1 tsp. of watermelon seed oil

- 1 tsp. of melon blossom oil

Steps

1. Melt the Shea butter, jojoba oil and coconut oil over medium heat in a saucepan. Remove from heat once they've melded together.

2. Pour the watermelon seed oil and melon blossom oil into this mixture and mix thoroughly.

3. Pour into jars and let it set.

4. Use within a couple of months.

Honey Massage Body Butter

Ingredients

- 1 cup of cocoa butter

- 1 cup of Shea butter

- 3 tbsp. of apricot kernel oil

- 1/3 tbsp. of vitamin E oil

- 2 tbsp. of honey powder

Steps

1. Use a double broiler to melt the cocoa and Shea butter over low heat. Keep stirring for about 20 minutes till they are completely melted together.

2. Remove the melted butters from heat and pour into a bowl. Add the apricot kernel, vitamin E and honey powder to this. Stir it all together.

3. Whip the mixture using a hand mixer to get a frosting-like consistency. It should become light and fluffy by the time you are done. While doing the whipping, place the bowl in some cold water so that it cools down.

4. Now scoop the body butter into glass jars and store in a cool place when you aren't using them.

Rose and Lavender Body Butter

Ingredients

- 8 drops of lavender essential oil

- 8 drops of rose essential oil

- 2 drops of rose geranium oil

- 1 cup of cocoa butter

- 1 cup of Shea butter

- 2 tbsp. of jojoba oil

- 1/3 tsp. of vitamin E oil

Steps

1. Melt the cocoa butter and Shea butter in a bowl over a pot of hot water. The heat should be on the low setting.

2. Take the bowl off the heat once the ingredients are completely melted together.

3. Now add the lavender, rose and rose geranium oils and stir. Then add the jojoba oil with vitamin E and continue to stir.

4. Place this bowl in a pan of cold water and hold it firmly. Now use a hand mixer to whip it into a smooth consistency. Keep whipping till small peaks form, like

whipped cream.

5. Scoop the body butter into containers and use as you please.

Cheerful Summer Body Butter

Ingredients

- 8 drops of orange essential oil

- 4 drops of ylang ylang essential oil

- 5 drops of grapefruit essential oil

- 2 drops of rose geranium essential oil

- ¾ cup of cocoa butter

- 1 cup of Shea butter

- ¼ tsp. of vitamin E oil

- 2 tbsp. of jojoba oil

Steps

1. Place a wide pot filled halfway with water

over low heat. Put a bowl inside it and put the cocoa and Shea butter into the bowl.

2. Melt the butters and then take the bowl off the heat.

3. Add the orange, ylang ylang, grapefruit and rose geranium essential oils into this butter and stir together thoroughly.

4. Then add the vitamin E and jojoba oil.

5. Now place the bowl with the mixture in a pan of cold water. Hold it in place and whip the mixture together using a hand mixer.

6. Keep whipping the body butter till you get a whipped-cream-like consistency and it is cool.

7. Now store this body butter in jars in a cool, dark place till you want to use it.

Raspberry and Vanilla Body Butter

Ingredients

- ¾ cup of cocoa butter

- ¾ cup of Shea butter

- 5 drops of grape seed oil

- 2 tbsp. of apricot kernel oil

- 2 tsp. of vitamin E oil

- 8 drops of black raspberry fragrance oil

- 5 drops of vanilla oil

Steps

1. Use a double boiler to melt the Shea and cocoa butter together over low heat; add the grape seed oil and apricot kernel oil into this bowl.

2. Remove the mixture from heat and add

the vitamin E, black raspberry with and oil. Stir it all together.

3. Place the bowl in a pan of cold water and let it cool down.

4. After about 15 minutes use a hand mixer to whip this mixture. Do this twice more at 15-minute intervals. The mixture should have a whipped-cream-like consistency. Small peaks should appear as you whip it well.

5. Then spoon this delicious-smelling body butter into glass jars for storage. Keep it in a cool place so that the butter remains thick, or it might melt in warm temperatures.

Arrowroot Body Butter

Ingredients

- 1/3 cup of Shea butter

- 1/3 cup of mango butter

- ½ cup of coconut oil

- 5 tbsp. of almond oil

- 5 tbsp. of hemp oil

- 5 tbsp. of olive oil

- 5 tbsp. of grape seed oil

- 2 tbsp. of arrowroot powder

- 1 tsp. of vitamin E oil

Steps

1. Use the double boiler method to melt the Shea butter, mango butter and coconut oil in a bowl. Perform this procedure over low heat so the mixture completely melts but doesn't boil.

2. Then remove the bowl from heat and let it cool for a while.

3. Add the arrowroot powder, vitamin E and

other oils into this bowl. Stir them together well.

4. Then use an electric hand mixer to whip the mixture into a smooth and fluffy consistency. Set it aside for a while and whisk it again till it looks like whipped cream.

5. Now scoop this body butter into jars and let them set overnight before using.

Hemp and Oat Body Butter Bar

Ingredients

- ½ cup of Shea butter

- 6 tbsp. of oat oil

- 6 tbsp. of hemp oil

- 1/3 cup of beeswax

Steps

1. Use the double boiler method to melt the Shea butter and beeswax. After a while add the oat oil and hemp oil as well. Melt these all over low heat.

2. Keep stirring for about 20 minutes.

3. Remove from heat and pour the mixture into a mould or tin to cool down and form a bar.

4. Store this in a cool place to keep the form.

Cherry Body Butter

Ingredients

- 1 cup of Shea butter

- ½ cup of coconut oil

- ½ cup of grape seed oil

- 4 tsp. of cherry extract

Steps

1. Place a pot filled halfway with water over low heat. Put the Shea butter and coconut oil in a bowl and place this over the pot. After a while add the grape seed oil. Keep it over heat for about 20 minutes or until everything has melted together.

2. Take the bowl off the heat and leave it aside or put it in the fridge to cool for a while.

3. Then use an electric hand mixer to whip it into a fluffy consistency. Add the cherry extract into it slowly as you are blending. The end product should look like peaky whipped cream.

4. Scoop this body butter into a jar and store in a cool place till you are ready to use it.

Avocado Body Butter

Ingredients

- 500 g of Shea butter

- 110 g of cocoa butter

- 1/3 cup of avocado oil

- 2 tbsp. of vegetable glycerin

Steps

1. Use the double boiler method to melt the Shea butter and cocoa butter together. Slowly add in the vegetable glycerin and avocado oil as well. Melt these over low heat.

2. Take the bowl off heat and stir it to prevent any chunks from forming. Then use an electric hand mixer to whip the body butter into a smooth and fluffy consistency.

3. Scoop it into jars and use as you need.

Lavender Body Butter

Ingredients

- 1 Vitamin E capsule

- 10 drops Lavender essential oil

- 2 tablespoons lanolin

- 3 tablespoons aloe vera gel

- 1 teaspoon honey

- 2 tablespoons beeswax

- 1 ½ tablespoons olive oil

- 4 tablespoons coconut oil

Steps

1. Heat all your oils, honey, and beeswax over medium heat in a double boiler.

2. Heat aloe over high heat in a separate double boiler until melted. Combine with the beeswax mixture and stir well.

3. Add in lanolin and stir until melted, then lower the heat. Stir in capsule together with the essential oils. Now whip the mixture to smoothness.

4. When done, transfer to jars and allow to cool.

Rosemary Mint Whipped Shea Body Butter

Ingredients

- 10 drops Rosemary Essential Oil

- 20 drops Spearmint Essential Oil

- 45 grams Kukui Nut Oil

- 90 grams Shea Butter

- 45 grams Cocoa Butter

Steps

1. Measure out cocoa butter and combine

with shea butter, before drizzling with Kukui Nut oil.

2. Put the bowl containing the mixture over a pan of simmering water, for the oils and butters to melt.

3. Cool the melted mixture for around 10 minutes, before refrigerating for about 20 minutes.

4. Using a whisk attachment, blend the mixture for around 15 minutes, and return to the freezer for an additional 15-20 minutes.

5. Then continue to whisk as the mixture turns creamy, and scrap down the sides of the bowl as required. You may return the mixture to the freezer to make it super cold.

6. Add in your essential oils and store.

Whipped Body Butter with Coconut Oil

Ingredients

- A few drops essential oils, any

- 1 teaspoon vitamin E oil

- 1 cup coconut oil

Steps

1. Into a mixing bowl, combine the coconut oil, vitamin E oil and few drops of essential oils.

2. Combine under high speed using a wire whisk for about 6-7 minutes. By now, the whipped butter should be of light and airy consistency.

3. Spoon the whipped coconut oil body butter into a container or glass jar and cover lightly.

4. Store the butter either at room temperature or under refrigeration to avoid melting of the oil.

Coconut Rose Body Butter

Ingredients

- 10 drops Rose essential oil

- 3 grams cornstarch

- 1 ml Alkanet infused oil

- 10 grams Jojoba oil

- 60 grams Coconut oil, refined

Steps

1. Into a glass bowl, combine cornstarch, Alkanet infused oil, Jojoba oil and coconut oil.

2. Over a pan that contains simmering water, heat the coconut oil to fully melt it

and then whisk to combine the ingredients properly. Allow the mixture to cool over room temperature.

3. After chilling, add in your essential oils and continue to whisk to form a fluffy substance that appears as frosting.

4. Spoon or pipe the mixture into a small jar and store at temperatures below 70 degrees. The butter should be used within 3 months.

Almond oil Body Butter

Ingredients

- ½ cup almond oil, melted

- ½ cup coconut oil

- 1 cup organic raw Shea butter

Steps

1. Melt the coconut oil and Shea butter into the top of a double boiler. When melted, remove from heat and then chill for around 30 minutes.

2. Add in almond oil, essential oils of choice and then stir to blend.

3. Freeze the oil mixture for some time, and allow the oils to partially solidify.

4. Then start to whip the mixture until you obtain a butter-like consistency.

5. You can then store the butter in a glass jar.

Super Glowy Body Butter

Ingredients

- 1 drop tea tree oil

- 7 ounces shea butter

- 2 cups organic coconut oil

- Essential oils like lavender, peppermint

Steps

1. To a double boiler or microwave, add in shea butter and coconut oil and melt the mixture. When melted, remove from heat, and pour in some tea tree oil and essential oils of choice.

2. Now blend the mixture for some few seconds, and then allow to cool until it solidifies. Alternatively, you can refrigerate the mixture.

3. Then whip the solid mixture until it turns smooth and fluffy, and pour into glass jar for storage.

Soothing Body Butter

Ingredients:

- 15-20 drops of tea tree oil

- Few drops of vitamin E

- 2 tablespoons jojoba oil

- 6 tablespoons cocoa butter

- ½ cup coconut oil

Steps

1. Into a glass container, melt some cocoa butter on a double boiler placed on a stove top or in an oven at low temperature.

2. Allow the cocoa butter to melt and then remove from heat. Add in jojoba oil, coconut oil and then stir to combine.

3. Allow the mixture to solidify within few hours or overnight, under ordinary temperatures. You may speed up the process by refrigerating.

4. Whip the solidified mixture using a stand mixer for 6-10 minutes on high speed,

and stop occasionally to stir down the sides as required.

5. Finally add in the tea tree oil and combine to mix. Store in glass jars.

Pretty in Pink Body Butter

Ingredients

- 5-10 drops essential oils

- 1-3 drops pink food dye

- 1 ½ cups vegetable shortening

- 1 cup coconut oil

Steps

1. Mix food dye, vegetable shortening, and coconut oil in a large bowl. Combine the mixture with an electric mixer to attain a pink whip.

2. Add 2 additional drops of food dye and other

essential oils, and then use a spatula to whip the butter to blend the ingredients.

3. Spoon the butter into glass jars.

DIY cranberry body butter

Ingredients:

- 1 drop orange essential oil

- 1 tablespoon cranberries, frozen

- 1 tablespoon shea butter

- ¼ cup coconut oil

Steps

1. Combine shea butter and coconut oil in a large bowl, and then combine using an electric mixer for about 5-8 minutes.

2. To your food processor, add in cranberries and pulse to attain tiny pieces.

3. Combine the pulsed cranberries in the coconut oil mixture, and put it through fine mesh sieve. Use a spatula to press the mixture through the mess into a bowl.

4. To the bowl, add in your favorite essential oil and use a spoon to mix.

5. Pour the mixture into a small jar and then close it. The butter can stay in your fridge for one week.

Coconut Vanilla Body Butter

Ingredients

- 1 (16 fluid ounces) jar of coconut oil

- 1 capful of vanilla extract

- Few drops of essential oil, optional

Steps

1. Scoop the coconut oil from the jar into a

mixing bowl. Using a stand mixer, whip the coconut oil for 2-4 minutes, then add in vanilla extract. You can add other essential oils if you don't like vanilla.

2. Continue to mix on high for about 5 minutes, while ensuring to scrap the sides of the bowl. When done, you'll have a fluffy lotion-like substance.

3. Now transfer into containers and enjoy your butter.

Vanilla Bean Body Butter

Ingredients:

1 vanilla bean

½ cup coconut oil

½ cup sweet almond oil

1 cup raw cocoa butter

Steps

1. Melt coconut oil and cocoa butter for a few seconds, and then remove from heat. Allow the mixture to cool for around 30 minutes.

2. Into a food processor or coffee grinder, process vanilla bean until fine.

3. Into the coconut oil and cocoa butter mixture, stir in the almond oil and vanilla and mix.

4. Freeze for around 20 minutes to chill completely, and oils to start to solidify.

5. Into a food processor or electric mixer, whip the contents to achieve a butter-like substance.

6. Spoon into containers or glass jars, and keep in the fridge.

Coffee Butter Foot Crème

Ingredients

- 0.2 ounces optiphen

- 5 ml peppermint essential oil

- 5 ml dark rich chocolate fragrance oil

- 15.6 ounces distilled water

- 1 ounce emulsifying wax

- 1.2 ounces stearic acid

- 2.4 ounces sunflower oil

- 3.1 ounces coffee butter

- 0.7 ounces white beeswax

Steps

1. Mix together sunflower oil, coffee butter, beeswax, Stearic acid and emulsifying wax in a heatproof container, as the waxes have high melting points.

2. Heat the distilled water in a separate heatproof container, to achieve high temperatures to sustain the melted beeswax. You need to maintain temperatures at 150-155 degrees.

3. Ensure that the temperatures of the oil mixture are within 5-10 degrees of the water. Add in the oils and mix for about 2-3 minutes.

4. Slightly cool the mixture and add in Optiphen, a preservative. Also add in peppermint and dark rich chocolate fragrance oil and blend for a minute.

5. Pour the mixture when it's warm, and wait for it to settle for about a day, before you put lids on. This allows enough time for the butter to cool, and to prevent any condensing in the containers.

Black Raspberry Vanilla Fragrance Butter

Ingredients

- 10 grams black raspberry vanilla

fragrance oil

- 4 grams vitamin E oil

- 65 grams apricot kernel oil

- 24 grams grape-seed oil

- 155 grams shea butter

- 156 grams cocoa butter

Steps

1. Weigh out the appropriate amounts of apricot kernel oil, grape-seed oil and butters and use your double boiler to melt them. Heat the mixture to completely melt, ensuring you don't make the oils too.

2. Now remove the melted mixture and then pour in black raspberry vanilla fragrance oil and vitamin E oil. Stir to mix.

3. Transfer the mixture into a mixing bowl and then set over another bowl that is full

of ice to chill. You can as well cover and keep in the freezer.

4. Allow the mixture to thicken, and keep on whipping at regular intervals of about 20 minutes. To facilitate cooling and thickening, keep the mixture over ice bowl or in the refrigerator. Every time you mix, the mixture will thicken into whipped butter consistency.

5. When your butter solidifies, just spoon into jars.

Edible Chocolate Body Butter

Ingredients

- ¼ cup cacao powder

- ½ tablespoon vanilla powder

- 1/3 cup agave nectar

- ¾ cup coconut oil, melted

Optional Add-ons

- ½ teaspoon lavender flowers, powdered

- 1-2 drops rose essential oil

- 1 teaspoon maca

- ½ teaspoon cistanche

Steps

1. Into a food processor, place cacao

   powder, vanilla powder, agave nectar, coconut oil and add-ons and blend to mix them.

2. Transfer to small jars and store in the fridge to set. You may also keep at a cool place to allow the butter to solidify.

Homemade Body Butter

Ingredients

- 7 drops lavender essential oil

- 7 drops lime essential oil

- 1 ml vitamin E (or 1 capsule)

- Dried rose petals, fresh rosemary

- 1 tablespoon olive oil

- 1 tablespoon coconut oil, mint infused

- 2 tablespoons solid shea butter

Steps

1. Into a double boiler, melt coconut oil and shea butter.

2. Pour in vegetable oil and dried or fresh herbs. In case you use herbs, just heat the mixture for 20 minutes, strain gently, and then squeeze out all the oil from your herbs.

3. When done, remove from heat and allow to cool, to about 30 degrees Celsius or

cooler. Now add vitamin E and your essential oils.

4. Whip the butter to achieve a thick and fluffy substance, for about 5-10 minutes. If the butter does not tend to get ready, trying cooling until it turns to become solid. Then start to whip again.

5. Use a spoon or spatula to scoop the butter into jars.

Frankincense Whipped Body Butter

Ingredients

- 30 drops Sacred Frankincense essential oil

- 1 teaspoon Vitamin E

- 1 ounce raw organic cocoa butter

- ½ cup mango butter

- ½ cup shea butter

- ½ cup organic, virgin coconut oil

Steps

1. Combine cocoa butter, mango butter, and shea butter in a double boiler and allow the mixture to melt.

2. Transfer the mixture to a heat-safe container or stainless steel. Then stir in the coconut oil and allow it to melt.

3. Let the mixture to rest and chill for about 45 minutes, until the bowl is safe to touch.

4. Add in Sacred Frankincense essential oil and vitamin E to the cool mixture, and cover.

5. Keep in the fridge for around 40 minutes, to allow the mixture to firm up. The mixture should not solidify.

6. Whip the semi-solid mixture using a

hand mixture, until some fluffy peaks start to form. Scoop the butter into glass jar.

DIY Body Butter

Ingredients

- 50 drops of vanilla essential oil

- 1 teaspoon of Vitamin E oil

- ½ cup of coconut oil

- 1 cup of shea butter

Steps

1. Into a medium sized container, pour vanilla essential oil, vitamin E oil, coconut oil and shea butter.

2. Mix the ingredients for about 5-7 minutes, to form a light and fluffy substance.

3. Transfer the butter into a Mason jar or other glass container and store. Ensure to keep the butter away from extreme temperatures.

Eucalyptus Whipped Body Butter

Ingredients

- 3 drops peppermint essential oil

- 10 drops eucalyptus essential oil

- 1½ teaspoons castor oil

- 1 tablespoon carrier oil

- 6 tablespoons cocoa butter

- 6 tablespoons shea butter

- ½ cup coconut oil

Steps

1. Warm cocoa butter, shea butter and

coconut oil over very low heat in a double boiler. When softened, pour into a medium bowl.

2. Add in peppermint essential oil, eucalyptus essential oil, castor oil, and carrier oil and stir together. Put the container with the mixture into the fridge until the oils become soft and thick.

3. Allow the mixture to firm but not solidify, and then remove from the fridge. Use a stand mixer or hand beaters to whip the mixture, to form a light and fluffy substance.

4. Scoop the butter into glass jars and keep sealed.

Lime Whipped Coconut Oil

Ingredients

- 20 drops lemon essential oil

- 20 drops lime essential oil

- 2 tablespoons aloe vera gel

- 1 tablespoon olive oil, macadamia nut oil or castor oil

- ½ cup coconut oil

Steps

1. Into a mixing bowl, put the essential oils, aloe Vera gel, olive oil, and coconut oil without melting the coconut oil. The oil best whips in solid form.

2. On high speed, beat with an electric mixer using a wire whisk attachment for about 3-7 minutes. Whip until you obtain a soft and fluffy consistency.

3. Use a spatula or a spoon to transfer the whipped body butter into glass jar and seal. The butter can stay at room temperature or in the fridge in case the house is warm.

Sugar Cookie Whipped Body Butter

Ingredients

- 10 grams sugar cookies fragrance oil

- 4 grams Vitamin E oil

- 52 grams fractionated coconut oil

- 48 grams Argan oil

- 100 grams Shea butter

- 100 grams mango butter

- 100 grams cocoa butter

Steps

1. Weigh out the butters, coconut oil and Argan oil. Into a double boiler, melt the oils and butters until fully melted.

2. Once melted, remove from heat and add in sugar cookies fragrance oil and vitamin E oil and stir.

3. Transfer the mixture into a mixing bowl, cover and cool in the fridge. Alternatively, you may set on a different bowl that is full of ice to chill faster.

4. Allow the mixture to thicken, and then start to whip in intervals of 20 minutes, using a hand mixer. Whip the butter for some few minutes.

5. To allow thickening or cooling, return the mixture to the ice bowl or fridge and continue to mix to form the whipped butter.

6. Allow the butter to solidify and then spoon into 4-ounce mason jars and store.

Healing Body Butter

Ingredients

- 20 drops vanilla extract

- 10 drops frankincense

- 10ml Rosehip oil

- 5mls 100% Argan oil

- ½ cup shea butter

- ½ cup cocoa butter

Steps

1. Melt the Shea butter and cocoa butter over double boiler.

2. Add in vanilla extract, frankincense, rosehip, and Argan oil. Into a food processor or other mixer, whip the oils and the essential oils to obtain butter.

3. When done, pour the butter into glass jars or tub, and then store into the fridge. The healing butter is best used after shower.

Lavender Vanilla Body Butter

Ingredients

- 4-8 drops carrot seed essential oil

- 15-20 drops of lavender essential oil

- 25-30 drops of vanilla essential oil

- 1 teaspoon red raspberry seed oil

- 1/8 cup avocado oil

- ¼ cup coconut oil

- ¼ cup mango butter

Steps

1. Melt avocado oil, coconut oil and mango butter over low heat in a double boiler. You may use a whisk to mix the oils.

2. When melted, remove from heat and allow to cool for several minutes. Add in red raspberry seed oil, and transfer the bowl with the mixture to a freezer.

3. Allow the mixture to cool to have the liquid set up, though soft for whipping.

4. Remove the mixture from the freezer or fridge and then add in the essential oils. Use a hand mixer or stand mixer to whip until you get a soft and airy consistency. In case the butter doesn't whip, return to the freezer and allow to cool for few minutes.

5. Store the butter in an airtight glass jar.

Sweet Citrus Vanilla Body Butter

Ingredients

- 10 drops lemon essential oil

- 15 drops of tangerine essential oil

- 15 drops of sweet orange essential oil

- 25-30 drops of vanilla essential oil

- 1 teaspoon red raspberry seed oil

- 1/8 cup jojoba oil or avocado oil

- ¼ cup coconut oil, virgin or refined

- ¼ cup kokum butter

Steps

1. Into a small sauce pan or double boiler over low heat, melt avocado oil, coconut oil and kokum butter. You may also use a whisk to combine the oils.

2. Once melted, remove the mixture from heat and allow it to cool for several minutes. Pour in the red raspberry seed oil and transfer into a freezer or fridge.

3. Allow the mixture to start solidifying, and then remove from the freezer or fridge, and add in the essential oils.

4. Whip the mixture using a hand mixer or stand mixer to obtain a soft and fluffy substance. If needed, return to the freezer to facilitate whipping.

5. Spoon the butter into glass jars and store.

White Chocolate Body Butter

Ingredients

- 10-15 drops of peppermint essential oil

- 1 teaspoon red raspberry seed oil

- 1/8 cup avocado oil

- ¼ cup coconut oil, virgin or refined

- ¼ cup cocoa butter

Steps

1. Over very low heat, melt avocado oil, coconut oil and cocoa butter in a small sauce pan or double boiler. Alternatively, use your whisk to have the oils combine together.

2. Once melted, remove the mixture from heat and allow to chill for some time. Add in a teaspoon of red raspberry and keep in a freezer.

3. Allow the mixture to chill and soften to facilitate whipping. The oils should now begin to thicken and turn whitish in color.

4. Remove from the freezer or fridge and add in the peppermint essential oil, and whip the mixture using a hand mixer or stand mixer. Allow a longer time in the freezer in case the butter doesn't whip properly.

5. When butter is ready, just spoon it into airtight jars and store under ordinary temperatures.

Citrus Body Butter

Ingredients

- 10 drops of citrus essential oil (like lemon)

- 2-3 tablespoons of distilled water

- 1 capsule of vitamin e oil

- ½ cup of grape-seed oil

- 2 tablespoons of beeswax

Steps

1. Mix together vitamin E, beeswax and grape-seed and heat to fully melt the beeswax. To do this, you can use a Pyrex bowl in the microwave or into a double boiler for 2 minutes.

2. Use a hand mixer to beat the oil mixture on high, and then add distilled water little by little. As the oil mixture turns milky, control the consistency by adding more distilled water.

3. After beating for 5 minutes, add about 10 drops of citrus oil preferably lemon, turn the mixer off and allow your butter to chill for 15-20 minutes.

4. Spoon into containers and store.

Eczema Relief Butter

Ingredients

- Few drops of vitamin E oil

- 5-10 drops cedar wood essential oil

- 10 drops lavender essential oil

- ¼ cup coconut oil

- ¼ cup shea butter

Steps

1. Combine shea butter and coconut oil using a stand mixer or bowl and then add in vitamin E and the essential oils.

2. Transfer the butter into a container or glass jar and store.

One-ingredient Body Butter

Ingredients

- 2 cups of shea butter

- Essential oil, optional

Steps

1. Melt the Shea butter in a double boiler. Store the melted butter in the fridge to facilitate firming up.

2. Add in 2-4 drops of your favorite essential oil

3. Use a hand held mixer or stand mixer to mix up until you get a semi-solid butter consisting of white peaks.

4. Now scoop the butter into jars and keep into a cool place.

Mint & Green Tea Whipped Body Butter

Ingredients

- 3-4 drops peppermint essential oil

- 8-9 fresh mint leaves, finely chopped

- ½ tablespoon Macha powder

- 7-8 drops Vitamin E

- 1 teaspoon olive oil

- ½ cup coconut oil

- ⅓ cup raw shea butter

Steps

1. Over medium heat, melt Shea butter and coconut oil on a stovetop and then add in olive oil. Transfer the melted butter into stainless steel or glass containers and store in the fridge.

2. Allow the mixture to rest and the oils to turn opaque. Put oils into the mixing bowl, place it on the stand mixer and then attach the whip.

3. Whip the oil mixture on high for about 3-

4 minutes, until you get a substance that looks like foamy egg white.

4. Remove from the mixer and keep in the fridge to make the oils solidify, for about 15 minutes.

5. Remove from the fridge and whip with the mixer on medium speed for a minute or so. Set the speed to high and whip for 3 additional minutes, until a creamy substance is formed.

6. Add in the mocha powder, vitamin E and the mint, and continue to whip for another 5 minutes, to form a whipped cream.

7. Scoop into glass jar and store in a cool place.

Tropical body butter

Ingredients

- 1/32nd teaspoon bronze mica

- 1g vitamin E

- 10g cocoa butter

- 10g virgin coconut oil

- 10g mango butter

Steps

1. Into a saucepan, melt vitamin E, cocoa butter, coconut oil and mango butter.

2. Stir and allow the molten mixture to cool, until an opaque mixture is formed, and then stir in bronze mica.

3. Pour the mixture into a container or tin and allow to cool.

All Natural Belly Butter

Ingredients

- 35 drops pure tangerine essential oil

- 1 tablespoon of vitamin E

- 3 tablespoons cocoa butter

- 3 tablespoons Shea butter

Steps

1. Melt shea butter, cocoa butter, vitamin E and tangerine essential oil in a double boiler. You can also melt on a stainless steel bowl that is placed over simmering water.

2. Use a mixing rod to stir the ingredients and allow them to blend.

3. Pour the hot liquid carefully into preferred container and allow to cool.

Whipped peppermint bark body butter

Ingredients

- ¼ teaspoon peppermint extract

- 2 tablespoon vitamin E oil

- ¼ cup coconut oil

- ¼ cup shea butter

- ¼ cup cocoa butter

Steps

1. Melt Vitamin E oil, coconut oil, Shea butter and cocoa butter in a heat-proof bowl for about 3 minutes. Continue to stir for all oils to melt and blend.

2. Stir in the peppermint extract and keep the mixture in a freezer for about 15-20 minutes. The oil should begin to get firm but not solidify.

3. Pour the oils into the bowl of a stand mixer and whip for about 5-8 minutes. You can use an electric beater on high speed or with whisk attachment. Whip until a soft and fluffy substance is formed.

4. Ensure to scrap the sides using a rubber spatula at regular intervals of 2 minutes. Then scoop the bu

5. tter into a glass jar and keep at room temperature.

Whipped Tallow Body butter

Ingredients

- 2 teaspoons vitamin E oil

- 1 teaspoon peppermint essential oil

- ½ cup of jojoba oil

- ½ cup tallow

- ½ cup shea butter

Steps

1. Using a glass bowl over a pot of simmering water or a double boiler, heat the tallow and shea butter gently until they melt.

2. Remove the bowl from heat then stir in the jojoba oil. Let it chill for about five minutes in an ice bath then stir in the Vitamin E oil and peppermint essential oil

3. Using a hand mixer or stand mixer, whip the body butter until stiff peaks form.

4. Scoop the mixture into glass jars and keep away from direct sunlight.

The Basic Process

If you want to get directly into inventing your own recipes and have already chosen ingredients for your body butter, remember the steps of the process:

1. Melt solid ingredients first (butters, oils that are solid at room temperature, beeswax) on very low heat.

2. Add liquid oils. Stir to combine well and make a smooth mass.

3. Remove from heat and add other ingredients, like essential oils, aloe vera gel etc.

4. Let mixture cool. If desired, whip using a mixer.

Another option is simply mixing ingredients with soft and liquid consistency – those that don't have to be melted to blend with other ingredients – and using them as your body butters. That's really easy!

Chapter 8: How To Apply Body Butter

1. The best time to apply your body butter is after a bath or shower. Pat yourself dry with a clean towel, but leave your skin a little moist so that the butter is absorbed better. It is best applied at night due to its thick consistency. It may feel a little too heavy if you apply it during the day.

2. As body butters are a little greasy, use just a dollop, not too much. Rub it into your skin with gentle yet firm strokes. Keep massaging it in till it is fully absorbed by your body.

3. Areas, which get especially dry (like your feet, elbows, etc.) should be given more attention. Use two coats of butter on such areas if you think it is necessary.

4. For overnight moisturizing, apply the body butter on your hands and feet after soaking them in warm water and then sleep with some gloves or socks on. When you wake up and remove them, your skin will feel extremely soft. This is really helpful during the winter, when your skin tends to get dry or cracked.

5. You need not apply them every day; a couple of times a week will do wonders for your skin. You can do an exfoliating and moisturizing routine by yourself at home whenever you get the chance.

6. Apply the body butter onto your skin in the following ways for best results:

   - For your legs, take generous amounts of the body butter and apply in vigorous strokes, going up and down at first and then only upward. This will tone your skin better. Rub around your knees in a circular motion.

- Stroke the body butter onto your arms in an up-and-down motion with firm strokes. Be rigorous and apply all over, around your shoulders as well as your armpits.

- For your neck and chest area, use gentle strokes to apply the butter.

- Apply around your stomach in circular motion. Massage your sides in upward strokes to lift the skin up.

- Apply the cream onto your back using the opposite hand to reach the opposite side better on the upper back. It is much easier to apply the butter on the lower back.

These tips will help you get the most out of your body butter. It is important to apply the body butter in the correct way to get smooth and supple skin which does not sag but is tight and firm. Proper application will also prevent the appearance of unwanted stretch marks on your body.

How does body butter help?

1. Dry patches- our skin tends to get dry patches, especially around the elbows and knees. Massaging a little body butter into these areas will prevent dry, flaky skin and make it smooth.

2. Hand and Foot care- it is important to pay attention to your hands and feet on a regular basis. A little is enough to moisturize both hands. For best results on your feet, soak them in warm water and scrub off any dry skin. Apply the body butter onto your feet and put on your socks for overnight moisturizing.

3. Makeup remover- Body butter is also useful

for removing makeup at the end of the day. Just put a little on a cotton swab and swipe it over your skin. It easily removes mascara as well.

4. Moisturizing face- Body butters are more suitable for dry or mature skin on the face. Just rub some onto your hands and apply on your face in firm, broad strokes. Do the same over your neck. Don't apply too much or your face will end up feeling greasy.

5. Aftershave lotion- Skin needs better care after shaving or any hair removal. Massage some of the body butter into the shaved areas to prevent scaly skin and give it a smooth finish.

6. Massage- you can use some body butter instead of massage oils. It will slide over your skin, leaving it smooth and silky. You can make different combinations of body butter for this purpose.

Enjoy the process of creating these and other body butters for a healthy, glowing and well-nurtured skin. Keep this book for reference and inspiration in creating your own body butters!

Conclusion

Thank you again for downloading this book!

I hope this book was able to give you a comprehensive insight into the world of body butters, and enough of information to start making your own 100% natural skincare products in the comfort of your own home.

If you still haven't decided what your next small DIY project will be, the next step is to choose your body butter recipe, pick some natural ingredients and get into the kitchen-laboratory. Just a few minutes in the kitchen and you can create marvelous, health-supporting body butters that will take deep care of your skin, keeping it hydrated, nurtured and young. It's a truly enjoyable way to take care of your skin!

Key Takeaways from This Book

- Body butters are nurturing, softening skin moisturizers and protectors with healing properties. They are made of only natural ingredients, combining together fruit, seed and nut oils and butters with essential oils, beeswax and other ingredients.

- Many commercially produced skincare products contain toxic chemical ingredients that block pores and can actually harm the health of skin and destroy its natural balance. This is one of the main reasons to make your own skincare products.

- If you know your skin type and the needs of your skin, you can combine natural ingredients to create your own healing body butters that are exactly suitable for your skin.

- To have a healthy, glowing skin, it's essential to take good care of your skin daily, but also make sure you don't overdo the cleanliness and decrease the skin's natural protection.

- Body butters can successfully become a part of your daily skincare routine as they are the best skin moisturizers, but you don't necessarily have to use them every single day.

- The main equipment for creating body butters at home is a stove, heatproof bowls, measuring cups and storage containers. Glass jars or containers with tight lids are the best option for storing body butters.

- As body butter consistency is pretty thick, many of them are prepared using a mixer. Whipping body butters give them a light and airy consistency.

- Body butter base ingredients are oils and butters. Sometimes, herb-infused oils can be used as base ingredients. You can prepare herb-infused oils at home to add healing herb properties and aromas to oils.

- Beeswax, honey, aloe vera gel, vitamin E oil, essential oils and other natural ingredients can be added to butter bases to change the consistency, add aromas, and increase healing properties of body butters.

- There are thousands of homemade body butter recipes, but that doesn't mean that you have to follow any of them. You can also create your own body butter recipes by combining ingredients that are perfectly suitable for your skin.

How to Put This Information into Action

If you've decided to start making your own body butters at home, first go through your kitchen and make sure you have all the <u>equipment</u> you'll need. Go ahead and purchase any you don't already have. Before buying your ingredients, you'll want to think about your skin type and any specific skin conditions or problems you may have, so take some time to review <u>Chapter 2</u> at this point. Then go through Chapters <u>4</u>, <u>5</u> and <u>6</u> to decide what butters and oils will do you the most good. Once you've decided on and acquired some appropriate ingredients, choose a recipe that uses them from <u>Chapter 7</u>, or follow the instructions for creating one of your own. Store your body butter in a cool place and refer to <u>Chapter 8</u> for the best ways to apply it to your skin.

Resources for Further Viewing and Reading

http://www.healthguidance.org/entry/5119/1/Toxic-Ingredients-in-Cosmetics-and-Skin-Care-Products.html

http://www.wisegeek.com/what-is-body-butter.htm

http://www.skinsight.com/diseaseGroups/obesity.htm

http://www.ncbi.nlm.nih.gov/pubmedhealth/PMH0005206/

http://www.webmd.com/beauty/wrinkles/cosmetic-procedures-overview-skin

http://health.howstuffworks.com/skin-care/daily/regimen

http://www.ingredientstodiefor.com/

http://www.makingcosmetics.com/

http://www.aromaweb.com/articles/whatinfu.asp

http://www.organicfacts.net/organic-oils/natural-essential-oils/list-of-essential-oils.html

http://health.howstuffworks.com/wellness/natural-medicine/herbal-remedies/amazing-aloe-vera.htm

http://apps.who.int/medicinedocs/en/d/Js2200e/6.html

http://www.livestrong.com/article/192009-skin-benefits-of-beeswax/

http://www.honeyhousenaturals.com/resources.php

http://www.livestrong.com/article/25515-benefits-vitamin-e-oil-skin/

http://modernhippiehousewife.com/

http://www.naturalandhealthyliving.com/top-12-best-diy-body-butter-recipes/

www.ingramcontent.com/pod-product-compliance
Lightning Source LLC
Chambersburg PA
CBHW070113030426
42335CB00016B/2138